SMOOTHIES FOR KIDNEY HEALTH

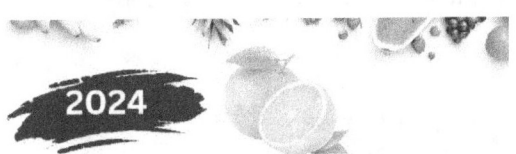

2024

SMOOTHIES FOR KIDNEY HEALTH

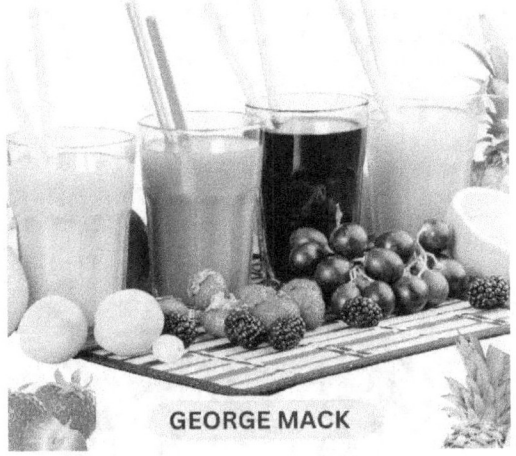

GEORGE MACK

GEORGE MACK

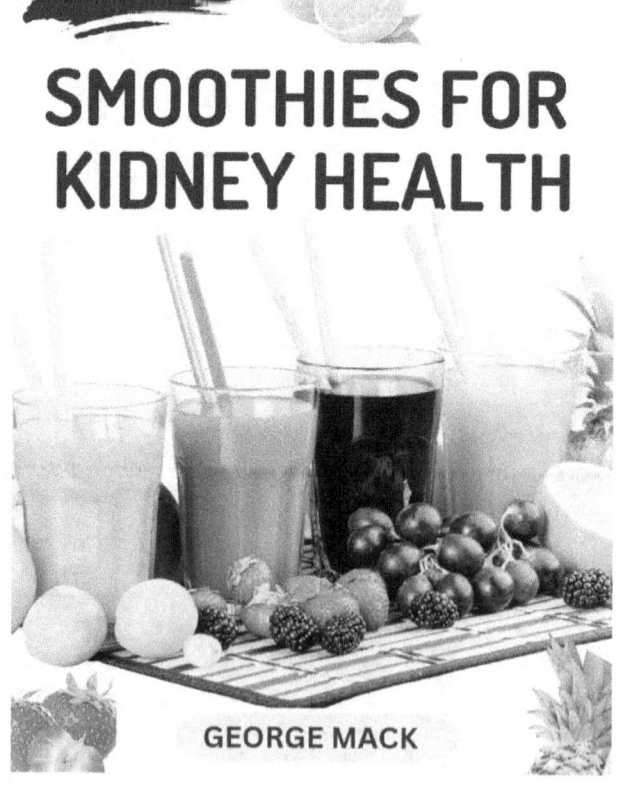

TABLE OF CONTENT

INTRODUCTION

Smoothies have gained popularity as a convenient and tasty way to incorporate essential nutrients into one's diet. For individuals with kidney health concerns, smoothies can serve as a particularly beneficial tool in managing their nutritional intake while supporting kidney function.

Kidney health is paramount for overall well-being, as these vital organs are responsible for filtering waste products and excess fluids from the bloodstream, regulating blood pressure, and maintaining electrolyte balance. When crafting smoothies for kidney health, it's essential to focus on ingredients that are kidney-friendly and supportive of renal function.

This means selecting ingredients that are low in sodium, potassium, and phosphorus while being rich in essential vitamins, minerals, and antioxidants. Incorporating fruits and vegetables that are lower in these minerals can help maintain a kidney-friendly diet.

Key ingredients for kidney-friendly smoothies include berries such as strawberries, blueberries, and raspberries, which are low in potassium and packed with antioxidants that may help protect against kidney damage. Leafy greens like spinach and kale provide an abundance of essential nutrients such as vitamin K, vitamin C, and folate, without contributing significantly to potassium levels.

Moreover, incorporating ingredients like Greek yogurt or almond milk can add creaminess and protein to smoothies while keeping phosphorus levels in check.

Adding a source of healthy fats such as avocado or flaxseed oil can provide additional nutrients and promote satiety.

Herbs and spices such as ginger, cinnamon, and turmeric not only enhance the flavor of smoothies but also offer anti-inflammatory properties that may benefit kidney health by reducing inflammation in the body.

However, it's crucial to be mindful of portion sizes and to consult with a healthcare professional or registered dietitian, especially for individuals with specific dietary restrictions or advanced kidney disease.

Additionally, monitoring overall nutrient intake, including protein, carbohydrates, and fats, is essential for maintaining a balanced diet and supporting kidney function.

incorporating kidney-friendly smoothies into one's diet can be a delicious and practical way to support overall kidney health while enjoying a variety of nutritious ingredients that promote well-being. By choosing the right ingredients and maintaining balance, smoothies can be a valuable addition to a kidney-friendly lifestyle.

CHAPTER ONE

Understanding Smoothies for Kidney Health

Smoothies tailored for kidney health are carefully crafted to support renal function and overall well-being.

Individuals with kidney concerns often need to manage their intake of certain minerals like potassium, phosphorus, and sodium, which can be achieved through mindful ingredient selection in smoothies.

Key considerations include choosing fruits and vegetables that are lower in potassium, such as berries, apples, and cucumbers, while limiting higher potassium options like bananas and oranges.

Similarly, selecting leafy greens like spinach and kale over higher phosphorus options helps maintain a kidney-friendly balance.

Incorporating sources of lean protein, such as Greek yogurt or almond milk, ensures a smoothie's nutritional profile while keeping phosphorus levels in check. Healthy fats from ingredients like avocado or flaxseed oil add richness and satiety without compromising kidney health.

Furthermore, incorporating herbs and spices like ginger and turmeric not only enhances flavor but also offers anti-inflammatory properties beneficial for kidney health.

Understanding the principles of creating kidney-friendly smoothies empowers individuals to make informed dietary choices that support renal function and overall health.

Consulting with a healthcare professional or registered dietitian can provide personalized guidance tailored to specific dietary needs and health goals.

Principles of Smoothies for Kidney Health

Moderation in Mineral Content: The primary principle of crafting smoothies for kidney health revolves around moderating the intake of minerals like potassium, phosphorus, and sodium. This involves selecting ingredients that are lower in these minerals to avoid burdening the kidneys.

Focus on Low-Potassium Ingredients: Potassium is a crucial electrolyte that needs to be managed carefully in kidney health. Choosing fruits and vegetables that are lower in potassium, such as berries, apples, and cucumbers, helps maintain a kidney-friendly balance.

Limit High-Phosphorus Ingredients: Phosphorus is another mineral that individuals with kidney concerns need to monitor. Opting for leafy greens like spinach and kale over higher phosphorus options helps in controlling phosphorus levels in smoothies.

Lean Protein Sources: Incorporating sources of lean protein, such as Greek yogurt or almond milk, ensures that smoothies provide essential nutrients without overloading on phosphorus.

Healthy Fats: Including healthy fats from ingredients like avocado or flaxseed oil adds richness and satiety to smoothies without compromising kidney health.

Anti-inflammatory Additions: Herbs and spices like ginger and turmeric not only enhance flavor but also offer anti-inflammatory properties beneficial for kidney health.

Consultation with Healthcare Professionals: It's crucial for individuals with kidney concerns to consult with healthcare professionals or registered dietitians to tailor smoothie recipes according to their specific dietary needs and health goals.

This ensures that smoothies are not only delicious but also supportive of renal function and overall well-being.

Benefits of Smoothies for Kidney Health

Smoothies offer a plethora of benefits for kidney health, making them a valuable addition to the diet of individuals managing renal concerns:

Nutrient Density: Smoothies can be packed with essential nutrients like vitamins, minerals, and antioxidants, which are vital for supporting overall health and kidney function.

By carefully selecting kidney-friendly ingredients, smoothies provide a concentrated source of nutrition.

Hydration: Adequate hydration is crucial for kidney health, as it helps to flush out toxins and waste products.

Smoothies, particularly those with high water content fruits and vegetables like cucumber and watermelon, contribute to hydration, supporting optimal kidney function.

Supports Electrolyte Balance: Smoothies can be tailored to help maintain electrolyte balance, essential for kidney health.

By incorporating ingredients with balanced levels of potassium, phosphorus, and sodium, smoothies can support the kidneys in maintaining proper electrolyte levels.

Easy to Digest: For individuals with kidney concerns who may experience digestive issues, smoothies offer a convenient and easily digestible option. Blending fruits and vegetables breaks down their fiber, making nutrients more readily available for absorption.

Weight Management: Maintaining a healthy weight is important for kidney health, and smoothies can be a helpful tool in weight management. They provide a satisfying and nutrient-dense option that can be incorporated into a balanced diet, supporting overall wellness and potentially aiding in weight control.

Convenient and Versatile: Smoothies are quick to prepare and can be customized according to taste preferences and dietary restrictions. This makes them a convenient option for individuals managing kidney health who may have specific dietary requirements.

Guidelines for Smoothies for Kidney Health:

Limit High-Potassium Ingredients: Choose fruits and vegetables that are lower in potassium, such as berries, apples, and cucumbers, to avoid overloading the kidneys with this mineral.

Manage Phosphorus Intake: Opt for leafy greens like spinach and kale over higher phosphorus options to help control phosphorus levels in smoothies.

Select Low-Sodium Options: Use unsalted or low-sodium ingredients to prevent excessive sodium intake, which can strain the kidneys.

Incorporate Lean Proteins: Include sources of lean protein like Greek yogurt, almond milk, or protein powder to support muscle health and satiety without adding excessive phosphorus.

Add Healthy Fats: Incorporate healthy fats from ingredients like avocado, flaxseed oil, or nuts to enhance flavor and provide essential fatty acids without compromising kidney health.

Choose Low-Sugar Options: Opt for naturally sweet ingredients like fruits instead of adding refined sugars or sweetened syrups to keep sugar levels in check.

Mindful Portion Control: Be mindful of portion sizes to avoid consuming excessive calories or nutrients, which can strain the kidneys.

Hydration: Use hydrating ingredients like water-rich fruits and vegetables to contribute to overall hydration, supporting kidney function

Consult with a Dietitian: Consider consulting with a registered dietitian who specializes in kidney health to create personalized smoothie recipes tailored to individual dietary needs and preferences.

Foods To Eat And Avoid for Smoothies for Kidney Health

When crafting smoothies for kidney health, it's important to carefully select ingredients that support renal function while avoiding those that may burden the kidneys. Here are some foods to incorporate and avoid:

- **Foods to Eat:**

Berries: Berries like strawberries, blueberries, and raspberries are low in potassium and high in antioxidants, making them excellent choices for kidney-friendly smoothies.

Apples: Apples are low in potassium and provide fiber, which can aid in digestion and overall health.

Cucumbers: Cucumbers have a high water content and are low in potassium, making them hydrating and kidney-friendly additions to smoothies.

Leafy Greens: Spinach, kale, and other leafy greens are rich in vitamins and minerals while being low in potassium and phosphorus, making them ideal for kidney health.

Greek Yogurt: Greek yogurt is a good source of protein and calcium, but be mindful of portion sizes to avoid excess phosphorus intake.

- **Foods to Avoid:**

Bananas: Bananas are high in potassium, which can be problematic for individuals with kidney concerns. Opt for lower potassium fruits like berries instead.

Oranges: Oranges and other citrus fruits are high in potassium and should be limited in kidney-friendly smoothies.

Avocado: While healthy in moderation, avocados are high in potassium and should be used sparingly in smoothies for individuals with kidney issues.

Dairy Milk: Regular dairy milk can be high in phosphorus, so opt for alternatives like almond milk or coconut milk instead.

Added Sugars: Avoid adding refined sugars or sweetened syrups to smoothies, as excessive sugar intake can be detrimental to kidney health.

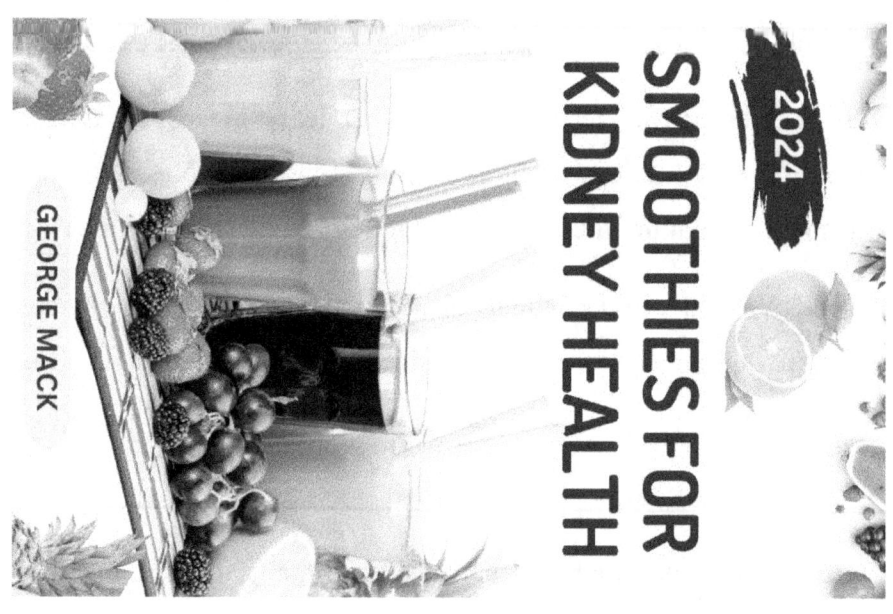

CHAPTER TWO

Smoothie Recipes for Kidney Health

1. Berry Citrus Delight Smoothie

Ingredients:

- 1/2 cup strawberries (sliced)
- 1/2 cup blueberries
- 1/2 cup raspberries
- 1/2 cup cucumber (peeled and sliced)
- 1/2 cup spinach leaves
- 1/2 cup Greek yogurt (unsweetened)
- 1 tablespoon chia seeds
- 1/2 teaspoon fresh ginger (grated)
- 1 cup coconut water (unsweetened)
- Ice cubes (optional)

Instructions:

1. Place strawberries, blueberries, raspberries, cucumber, spinach, Greek yogurt, chia seeds, and ginger in a blender.

2. Add coconut water to the blender for a hydrating base.

3. Blend on high speed until the mixture is smooth and well combined.

4. If desired, add ice cubes and blend again for a refreshing chill.

5. Pour the smoothie into a glass and enjoy this kidney-friendly, antioxidant-rich delight!

Preparation Time: Approximately 5-7 minutes

2. Green Protein Powerhouse Smoothie

Ingredients:

- 1/2 cup kale leaves (stems removed)
- 1/2 cup pineapple chunks (fresh or frozen)
- 1/2 banana (sliced, for creaminess)
- 1/2 cup cucumber (peeled and diced)
- 1/2 cup unsweetened almond milk
- 1/2 cup Greek yogurt (unsweetened)
- 1 tablespoon flaxseed meal
- 1 scoop protein powder (unflavored or vanilla)
- 1/2 teaspoon turmeric powder (optional for anti-inflammatory benefits)
- Ice cubes (optional)

Instructions:

1. Combine kale, pineapple, banana, cucumber, almond milk, Greek yogurt, flaxseed meal, protein powder, and turmeric in a blender.

2. Blend on high speed until all ingredients are well combined and the smoothie reaches a creamy consistency.

3. If desired, add ice cubes and blend again for a cool and refreshing texture.

4. Pour into a glass, and savor this protein-packed, kidney-friendly powerhouse!

Preparation Time: Approximately 6-8 minutes

3. Creamy Berry Blast Smoothie

Ingredients:

- 1/2 cup mixed berries (strawberries, blueberries, raspberries)
- 1/2 cup sliced peaches (fresh or frozen)
- 1/2 cup spinach leaves
- 1/2 cup Greek yogurt (unsweetened)
- 1 tablespoon almond butter (unsweetened)
- 1 tablespoon honey (optional, adjust to taste)
- 1/2 teaspoon vanilla extract
- 1/2 cup unsweetened almond milk
- Ice cubes (optional)

Instructions:

1. Place mixed berries, sliced peaches, spinach leaves, Greek yogurt, almond butter, honey (if using), and vanilla extract in a blender.

2. Add unsweetened almond milk to the blender for a creamy base.

3. Blend on high speed until all ingredients are well combined and the smoothie reaches a creamy consistency.

4. If desired, add ice cubes and blend again for a colder texture.

5. Pour into a glass, and indulge in this creamy and fruity delight that's gentle on the kidneys.

Preparation Time: Approximately 5-7 minutes

4. Tropical Turmeric Tango Smoothie

Ingredients:

- 1/2 cup pineapple chunks (fresh or frozen)
- 1/2 cup mango chunks (fresh or frozen)
- 1/2 cup spinach leaves
- 1/2 cup cucumber (peeled and diced)
- 1/2 cup coconut water (unsweetened)
- 1/2 cup Greek yogurt (unsweetened)
- 1 tablespoon chia seeds
- 1/2 teaspoon turmeric powder
- 1 teaspoon fresh lime juice
- Ice cubes (optional)

Instructions:

1. Combine pineapple chunks, mango chunks, spinach leaves, cucumber, coconut water, Greek yogurt, chia seeds, turmeric powder, and fresh lime juice in a blender.

2. Blend on high speed until all ingredients are well combined and the smoothie reaches a smooth consistency.

3. If desired, add ice cubes and blend again for a refreshing chill.

4. Pour into a glass, and revel in this tropical fusion with a hint of turmeric's anti-inflammatory goodness.

Preparation Time: Approximately 5-7 minutes

5. Refreshing Citrus Green Smoothie

Ingredients:

- 1/2 cup spinach leaves
- 1/2 cup kale leaves (stems removed)
- 1/2 cup cucumber (peeled and sliced)
- 1/2 cup pineapple chunks (fresh or frozen)
- 1/2 cup orange segments (fresh)
- 1/2 cup Greek yogurt (unsweetened)
- 1 tablespoon fresh mint leaves
- 1/2 cup coconut water (unsweetened)
- Ice cubes (optional)

Instructions:

1. In a blender, combine spinach leaves, kale leaves, cucumber slices, pineapple chunks, orange segments, Greek yogurt, and fresh mint leaves.
2. Pour in coconut water for added hydration and blend until smooth.
3. Add ice cubes if desired and blend again until well incorporated and chilled.
4. Serve immediately in a tall glass, and enjoy the refreshing taste of citrus combined with the nutritional goodness of greens.

Preparation Time: Approximately 5-7 minutes

6. Creamy Coconut Berry Smoothie Bowl

Ingredients:

- 1/2 cup mixed berries (strawberries, blueberries, raspberries)
- 1/2 cup sliced banana (fresh or frozen)
- 1/4 cup coconut milk (unsweetened)
- 1/4 cup Greek yogurt (unsweetened)
- 1 tablespoon unsweetened shredded coconut
- 1 tablespoon honey (optional, adjust to taste)

Toppings: Fresh berries, sliced banana, granola, additional shredded coconut.

Instructions:

1. In a blender, combine mixed berries, sliced banana, coconut milk, Greek yogurt, shredded coconut, and honey (if using).
2. Blend until smooth and creamy, adding more coconut milk if needed to reach desired consistency.
3. Pour the smoothie into a bowl and arrange toppings such as fresh berries, sliced banana, granola, and shredded coconut on top.
4. Serve immediately with a spoon and enjoy this creamy and nutritious smoothie bowl that's perfect for breakfast or a refreshing snack.

Preparation Time: Approximately 5-7 minutes

7. Tropical Green Smoothie with Mango

Ingredients:

- 1/2 cup spinach leaves
- 1/2 cup kale leaves (stems removed)
- 1/2 cup mango chunks (fresh or frozen)
- 1/2 cup pineapple chunks (fresh or frozen)
- 1/2 cup cucumber (peeled and sliced)
- 1/2 cup coconut water (unsweetened)
- 1/4 cup Greek yogurt (unsweetened)
- 1 tablespoon lime juice

- Ice cubes (optional)

Instructions:

1. Combine spinach leaves, kale leaves, mango chunks, pineapple chunks, cucumber slices, coconut water, Greek yogurt, and lime juice in a blender.
2. Blend on high speed until smooth and creamy, adding ice cubes if desired for a colder texture.
3. Once the desired consistency is reached, pour the smoothie into glasses and serve immediately.
4. Enjoy the refreshing and tropical flavors of this nutrient-packed green smoothie, perfect for supporting kidney health.

Preparation Time: Approximately 5-7 minutes

8. Peachy Protein Smoothie

Ingredients:

- 1/2 cup peaches (fresh or frozen, sliced)
- 1/2 cup strawberries (fresh or frozen)
- 1/2 cup cucumber (peeled and sliced)
- 1/2 cup Greek yogurt (unsweetened)
- 1 scoop unflavored or vanilla protein powder
- 1 tablespoon almond butter (unsweetened)
- 1 tablespoon honey (optional, adjust to taste)
- 1/2 cup unsweetened almond milk

- Ice cubes (optional)

Instructions:

1. In a blender, combine peaches, strawberries, cucumber slices, Greek yogurt, protein powder, almond butter, honey (if using), and unsweetened almond milk.
2. Blend until smooth and creamy, adjusting the consistency with additional almond milk if needed.
3. Add ice cubes if desired and blend again until well incorporated and chilled.
4. Pour the smoothie into glasses and serve immediately, savoring the sweet and creamy flavors of this peachy protein smoothie.

Preparation Time: Approximately 5-7 minutes

9. Blueberry Banana Bliss Smoothie

Ingredients:

- 1/2 cup blueberries (fresh or frozen)
- 1/2 banana (fresh or frozen, sliced)
- 1/2 cup spinach leaves
- 1/2 cup cucumber (peeled and sliced)
- 1/2 cup Greek yogurt (unsweetened)
- 1 tablespoon chia seeds
- 1 tablespoon honey (optional, adjust to taste)

- 1/2 cup unsweetened almond milk
- Ice cubes (optional)

Instructions:

1. Combine blueberries, banana slices, spinach leaves, cucumber slices, Greek yogurt, chia seeds, honey (if using), and unsweetened almond milk in a blender.
2. Blend until smooth and creamy, adjusting sweetness with honey if desired.
3. Add ice cubes if a colder texture is preferred and blend again until well mixed.
4. Pour the smoothie into glasses and serve immediately to enjoy the delightful blend of blueberries and banana with a hint of refreshing cucumber.

Preparation Time: Approximately 5-7 minutes

10. Mango Coconut Dream Smoothie

Ingredients:

- 1/2 cup mango chunks (fresh or frozen)
- 1/2 cup pineapple chunks (fresh or frozen)
- 1/4 cup Greek yogurt (unsweetened)
- 1/4 cup unsweetened coconut milk
- 1 tablespoon unsweetened shredded coconut
- 1 tablespoon honey (optional, adjust to taste)

- 1/2 cup coconut water (unsweetened)
- Ice cubes (optional)

Instructions:

1. In a blender, combine mango chunks, pineapple chunks, Greek yogurt, coconut milk, shredded coconut, honey (if using), and coconut water.
2. Blend until smooth and creamy, adjusting sweetness with honey if desired.
3. Add ice cubes if a colder texture is preferred and blend again until well mixed.
4. Pour the smoothie into glasses, garnish with additional shredded coconut if desired, and enjoy the tropical flavors of this mango coconut dream smoothie.

Preparation Time: Approximately 5-7 minutes

11. Kiwi Berry Blast Smoothie

Ingredients:

- 1 kiwi (peeled and sliced)
- 1/2 cup mixed berries (strawberries, blueberries, raspberries)
- 1/2 cup spinach leaves
- 1/2 cup cucumber (peeled and sliced)
- 1/2 cup Greek yogurt (unsweetened)
- 1 tablespoon honey (optional, adjust to taste)

- 1/2 cup coconut water (unsweetened)
- Ice cubes (optional)

Instructions:

1. Place kiwi slices, mixed berries, spinach leaves, cucumber slices, Greek yogurt, honey (if using), and coconut water in a blender.
2. Blend until smooth and creamy, adjusting sweetness with honey if desired.
3. Add ice cubes if a colder texture is preferred and blend again until well mixed.
4. Pour the smoothie into glasses, garnish with a kiwi slice if desired, and enjoy the refreshing and tangy flavors of this kiwi berry blast smoothie.

Preparation Time: Approximately 5-7 minutes

12. Apple Cinnamon Spice Smoothie

Ingredients:

- 1/2 apple (cored and sliced)
- 1/2 cup cucumber (peeled and sliced)
- 1/2 cup spinach leaves
- 1/2 teaspoon cinnamon powder
- 1/4 teaspoon nutmeg powder
- 1/2 cup Greek yogurt (unsweetened)

- 1 tablespoon honey (optional, adjust to taste)
- 1/2 cup unsweetened almond milk
- Ice cubes (optional)

Instructions:

1. Combine apple slices, cucumber slices, spinach leaves, cinnamon powder, nutmeg powder, Greek yogurt, honey (if using), and almond milk in a blender.
2. Blend until smooth and creamy, adjusting sweetness with honey if desired.
3. Add ice cubes if a colder texture is preferred and blend again until well mixed.
4. Pour the smoothie into glasses, sprinkle a dash of cinnamon on top if desired, and enjoy the comforting and aromatic flavors of this apple cinnamon spice smoothie.

Preparation Time: Approximately 5-7 minutes

13. Cherry Coconut Refresher Smoothie

Ingredients:

- 1/2 cup cherries (pitted, fresh or frozen)
- 1/2 cup pineapple chunks (fresh or frozen)
- 1/2 cup spinach leaves
- 1/2 cup cucumber (peeled and sliced)
- 1/2 cup Greek yogurt (unsweetened)

- 1 tablespoon unsweetened shredded coconut
- 1 tablespoon honey (optional, adjust to taste)
- 1/2 cup coconut water (unsweetened)
- Ice cubes (optional)

Instructions:

1. In a blender, combine cherries, pineapple chunks, spinach leaves, cucumber slices, Greek yogurt, shredded coconut, honey (if using), and coconut water.
2. Blend until smooth and creamy, adjusting sweetness with honey if desired.
3. Add ice cubes if a colder texture is preferred and blend again until well mixed.
4. Pour the smoothie into glasses, garnish with a sprinkle of shredded coconut if desired, and enjoy the tropical fusion of cherry and coconut flavors in this refreshing smoothie.

Preparation Time: Approximately 5-7 minutes

14. Lemon Blueberry Zest Smoothie

Ingredients:

- 1/2 cup blueberries (fresh or frozen)
- 1/2 banana (fresh or frozen, sliced)
- Zest of 1 lemon
- 1 tablespoon lemon juice

- 1/2 cup spinach leaves
- 1/2 cup Greek yogurt (unsweetened)
- 1 tablespoon honey (optional, adjust to taste)
- 1/2 cup unsweetened almond milk
- Ice cubes (optional)

Instructions:

1. Combine blueberries, banana slices, lemon zest, lemon juice, spinach leaves, Greek yogurt, honey (if using), and almond milk in a blender.
2. Blend until smooth and creamy, adjusting sweetness with honey if desired.
3. Add ice cubes if a colder texture is preferred and blend again until well mixed.
4. Pour the smoothie into glasses, garnish with a lemon slice or blueberries if desired, and enjoy the refreshing burst of lemon and blueberry flavors in this zesty smoothie.

Preparation Time: Approximately 5-7 minutes

15. Pineapple Mango Paradise Smoothie

Ingredients:

- 1/2 cup pineapple chunks (fresh or frozen)
- 1/2 cup mango chunks (fresh or frozen)
- 1/2 banana (fresh or frozen, sliced)

- 1/2 cup spinach leaves
- 1/2 cup Greek yogurt (unsweetened)
- 1 tablespoon chia seeds
- 1 tablespoon honey (optional, adjust to taste)
- 1/2 cup coconut water (unsweetened)
- Ice cubes (optional)

Instructions:

1. In a blender, combine pineapple chunks, mango chunks, banana slices, spinach leaves, Greek yogurt, chia seeds, honey (if using), and coconut water.
2. Blend until smooth and creamy, adjusting sweetness with honey if desired.
3. Add ice cubes if a colder texture is preferred and blend again until well mixed.
4. Pour the smoothie into glasses, garnish with a slice of pineapple or mango if desired, and enjoy the tropical paradise flavors of this refreshing smoothie.

Preparation Time: Approximately 5-7 minutes

16. Raspberry Lemonade Smoothie

Ingredients:

- 1/2 cup raspberries (fresh or frozen)
- Zest of 1 lemon

- 1 tablespoon lemon juice
- 1/2 cup cucumber (peeled and sliced)
- 1/2 cup Greek yogurt (unsweetened)
- 1 tablespoon honey (optional, adjust to taste)
- 1/2 cup coconut water (unsweetened)
- Ice cubes (optional)

Instructions:

1. Combine raspberries, lemon zest, lemon juice, cucumber slices, Greek yogurt, honey (if using), and coconut water in a blender.
2. Blend until smooth and creamy, adjusting sweetness with honey if desired.
3. Add ice cubes if a colder texture is preferred and blend again until well mixed.
4. Pour the smoothie into glasses, garnish with a lemon slice or fresh raspberries if desired, and enjoy the refreshing and tangy flavors of this raspberry lemonade smoothie.

Preparation Time: Approximately 5-7 minutes

17. Green Apple Kiwi Smoothie

Ingredients:

- 1 green apple (cored and sliced)
- 2 kiwis (peeled and sliced)

- 1/2 cup spinach leaves
- 1/2 cup cucumber (peeled and sliced)
- 1/2 cup Greek yogurt (unsweetened)
- 1 tablespoon honey (optional, adjust to taste)
- 1/2 cup coconut water (unsweetened)
- Ice cubes (optional)

Instructions:

1. Place green apple slices, kiwi slices, spinach leaves, cucumber slices, Greek yogurt, honey (if using), and coconut water in a blender.
2. Blend until smooth and creamy, adjusting sweetness with honey if desired.
3. Add ice cubes if a colder texture is preferred and blend again until well mixed.
4. Pour the smoothie into glasses, garnish with a slice of green apple or kiwi if desired, and enjoy the crisp and refreshing flavors of this green apple kiwi smoothie.

Preparation Time: Approximately 5-7 minutes

18. Banana Peach Cream Smoothie

Ingredients:

- 1/2 banana (fresh or frozen, sliced)
- 1 peach (pitted and sliced)

- 1/2 cup Greek yogurt (unsweetened)
- 1/4 cup coconut milk (unsweetened)
- 1 tablespoon unsweetened shredded coconut
- 1 tablespoon honey (optional, adjust to taste)
- Ice cubes (optional)

Instructions:

1. Combine banana slices, peach slices, Greek yogurt, coconut milk, shredded coconut, and honey (if using) in a blender.
2. Blend until smooth and creamy, adjusting sweetness with honey if desired.
3. Add ice cubes if a colder texture is preferred and blend again until well mixed.
4. Pour the smoothie into glasses, garnish with a sprinkle of shredded coconut if desired, and enjoy the creamy and tropical flavors of this banana peach cream smoothie.

Preparation Time: Approximately 5-7 minutes

19. Vanilla Berry Blast Smoothie

Ingredients:

- 1/2 cup mixed berries (strawberries, blueberries, raspberries)
- 1/2 cup spinach leaves
- 1/2 cup cucumber (peeled and sliced)
- 1/2 cup Greek yogurt (unsweetened)

- 1 tablespoon chia seeds
- 1 teaspoon vanilla extract
- 1 tablespoon honey (optional, adjust to taste)
- 1/2 cup unsweetened almond milk
- Ice cubes (optional)

Instructions:

1. In a blender, combine mixed berries, spinach leaves, cucumber slices, Greek yogurt, chia seeds, vanilla extract, honey (if using), and almond milk.
2. Blend until smooth and creamy, adjusting sweetness with honey if desired.
3. Add ice cubes if a colder texture is preferred and blend again until well mixed.
4. Pour the smoothie into glasses, garnish with a few whole berries if desired, and enjoy the delightful combination of vanilla and mixed berries in this refreshing smoothie.

Preparation Time: Approximately 5-7 minutes

20. Creamy Mango Banana Smoothie

Ingredients:

- 1/2 cup mango chunks (fresh or frozen)
- 1/2 banana (fresh or frozen, sliced)
- 1/2 cup spinach leaves

- 1/2 cup Greek yogurt (unsweetened)
- 1 tablespoon almond butter (unsweetened)
- 1 tablespoon honey (optional, adjust to taste)
- 1/2 cup unsweetened almond milk
- Ice cubes (optional)

Instructions:

1. Combine mango chunks, banana slices, spinach leaves, Greek yogurt, almond butter, honey (if using), and almond milk in a blender.
2. Blend until smooth and creamy, adjusting sweetness with honey if desired.
3. Add ice cubes if a colder texture is preferred and blend again until well mixed.
4. Pour the smoothie into glasses, garnish with a slice of mango or banana if desired, and enjoy the creamy and tropical flavors of this mango banana smoothie.

Preparation Time: Approximately 5-7 minutes

21. Creamy Pineapple Coconut Smoothie

Ingredients:

- 1/2 cup pineapple chunks (fresh or frozen)
- 1/2 banana (fresh or frozen, sliced)
- 1/4 cup Greek yogurt (unsweetened)

- 1/4 cup coconut milk (unsweetened)
- 1 tablespoon unsweetened shredded coconut
- 1 tablespoon honey (optional, adjust to taste)
- 1/2 cup unsweetened almond milk
- Ice cubes (optional)

Instructions:

1. In a blender, combine pineapple chunks, banana slices, Greek yogurt, coconut milk, shredded coconut, honey (if using), and almond milk.
2. Blend until smooth and creamy, adjusting sweetness with honey if desired.
3. Add ice cubes if a colder texture is preferred and blend again until well mixed.
4. Pour the smoothie into glasses, garnish with a sprinkle of shredded coconut if desired, and enjoy the tropical flavors of this creamy pineapple coconut smoothie.

Preparation Time: Approximately 5-7 minutes

22. Cherry Almond Bliss Smoothie

Ingredients:

- 1/2 cup cherries (pitted, fresh or frozen)
- 1/2 banana (fresh or frozen, sliced)
- 1/4 cup spinach leaves

- 1 tablespoon almond butter (unsweetened)
- 1 tablespoon honey (optional, adjust to taste)
- 1/2 teaspoon almond extract
- 1/2 cup unsweetened almond milk
- Ice cubes (optional)

Instructions:

1. Combine cherries, banana slices, spinach leaves, almond butter, honey (if using), almond extract, and almond milk in a blender.
2. Blend until smooth and creamy, adjusting sweetness with honey if desired.
3. Add ice cubes if a colder texture is preferred and blend again until well mixed.
4. Pour the smoothie into glasses, garnish with a cherry on top if desired, and enjoy the delicious blend of cherry and almond flavors in this refreshing smoothie.

Preparation Time: Approximately 5-7 minutes

23. Peachy Green Smoothie

Ingredients:

- 1/2 cup peaches (fresh or frozen, sliced)
- 1/2 cup pineapple chunks (fresh or frozen)
- 1/2 cup spinach leaves

- 1/2 cup cucumber (peeled and sliced)
- 1/2 cup Greek yogurt (unsweetened)
- 1 tablespoon honey (optional, adjust to taste)
- 1/2 cup coconut water (unsweetened)
- Ice cubes (optional)

Instructions:

1. Place peaches, pineapple chunks, spinach leaves, cucumber slices, Greek yogurt, honey (if using), and coconut water in a blender.
2. Blend until smooth and creamy, adjusting sweetness with honey if desired.
3. Add ice cubes if a colder texture is preferred and blend again until well mixed.
4. Pour the smoothie into glasses, garnish with a slice of peach or pineapple if desired, and enjoy the refreshing and fruity flavors of this peachy green smoothie.

Preparation Time: Approximately 5-7 minutes

24. Berry Avocado Dream Smoothie

Ingredients:

- 1/2 cup mixed berries (strawberries, blueberries, raspberries)
- 1/4 avocado (peeled and diced)
- 1/2 cup spinach leaves

- 1/2 cup Greek yogurt (unsweetened)
- 1 tablespoon honey (optional, adjust to taste)
- 1/2 cup unsweetened almond milk
- Ice cubes (optional)

Instructions:

1. In a blender, combine mixed berries, avocado chunks, spinach leaves, Greek yogurt, honey (if using), and almond milk.
2. Blend until smooth and creamy, adjusting sweetness with honey if desired.
3. Add ice cubes if a colder texture is preferred and blend again until well mixed.
4. Pour the smoothie into glasses, garnish with a few whole berries if desired, and enjoy the creamy and nutritious blend of berries and avocado in this dreamy smoothie.

Preparation Time: Approximately 5-7 minutes

25. Creamy Orange Mango Smoothie

Ingredients:

- 1/2 cup mango chunks (fresh or frozen)
- 1 orange (peeled and segmented)
- 1/2 cup Greek yogurt (unsweetened)
- 1 tablespoon honey (optional, adjust to taste)

- 1/2 cup unsweetened almond milk
- Ice cubes (optional)

Instructions:

1. In a blender, combine mango chunks, orange segments, Greek yogurt, honey (if using), and almond milk.
2. Blend until smooth and creamy, adjusting sweetness with honey if desired.
3. Add ice cubes if a colder texture is preferred and blend again until well mixed.
4. Pour the smoothie into glasses, garnish with an orange slice if desired, and enjoy the creamy and tropical flavors of this orange mango smoothie.

Preparation Time: Approximately 5-7 minutes

26. Kiwi Spinach Power Smoothie

Ingredients:

- 2 kiwis (peeled and sliced)
- 1/2 cup spinach leaves
- 1/2 cup cucumber (peeled and sliced)
- 1/2 cup pineapple chunks (fresh or frozen)
- 1/2 cup Greek yogurt (unsweetened)
- 1 tablespoon honey (optional, adjust to taste)
- 1/2 cup coconut water (unsweetened)

- Ice cubes (optional)

Instructions:

1. Place kiwi slices, spinach leaves, cucumber slices, pineapple chunks, Greek yogurt, honey (if using), and coconut water in a blender.
2. Blend until smooth and creamy, adjusting sweetness with honey if desired.
3. Add ice cubes if a colder texture is preferred and blend again until well mixed.
4. Pour the smoothie into glasses, garnish with a slice of kiwi if desired, and enjoy the energizing and nutrient-packed flavors of this kiwi spinach power smoothie.

Preparation Time: Approximately 5-7 minutes

27. Raspberry Beet Delight Smoothie

Ingredients:

- 1/2 cup raspberries (fresh or frozen)
- 1 small beet (cooked and peeled)
- 1/2 cup spinach leaves
- 1/2 cup Greek yogurt (unsweetened)
- 1 tablespoon honey (optional, adjust to taste)
- 1/2 cup unsweetened almond milk
- Ice cubes (optional)

Instructions:

1. In a blender, combine raspberries, cooked beet, spinach leaves, Greek yogurt, honey (if using), and almond milk.
2. Blend until smooth and creamy, adjusting sweetness with honey if desired.
3. Add ice cubes if a colder texture is preferred and blend again until well mixed.
4. Pour the smoothie into glasses, garnish with a few fresh raspberries if desired, and enjoy the vibrant and nutritious flavors of this raspberry beet delight smoothie.

Preparation Time: Approximately 5-7 minutes

28. Pineapple Turmeric Sunshine Smoothie

Ingredients:

- 1/2 cup pineapple chunks (fresh or frozen)
- 1/2 banana (fresh or frozen, sliced)
- 1/2 teaspoon turmeric powder
- 1/2 cup Greek yogurt (unsweetened)
- 1 tablespoon honey (optional, adjust to taste)
- 1/2 cup unsweetened almond milk
- Ice cubes (optional)

Instructions:

1. Combine pineapple chunks, banana slices, turmeric powder, Greek yogurt, honey (if using), and almond milk in a blender.

2. Blend until smooth and creamy, adjusting sweetness with honey if desired.

3. Add ice cubes if a colder texture is preferred and blend again until well mixed.

4. Pour the smoothie into glasses, garnish with a sprinkle of turmeric powder if desired, and enjoy the tropical and anti-inflammatory goodness of this pineapple turmeric sunshine smoothie.

Preparation Time: Approximately 5-7 minutes

29. Berry Spinach Protein Smoothie

Ingredients:

- 1/2 cup mixed berries (strawberries, blueberries, raspberries)
- 1/2 cup spinach leaves
- 1/2 banana (fresh or frozen, sliced)
- 1/2 cup Greek yogurt (unsweetened)
- 1 scoop vanilla protein powder
- 1 tablespoon chia seeds
- 1 tablespoon honey (optional, adjust to taste)

- 1/2 cup unsweetened almond milk
- Ice cubes (optional)

Instructions:

1. In a blender, combine mixed berries, spinach leaves, banana slices, Greek yogurt, protein powder, chia seeds, honey (if using), and almond milk.
2. Blend until smooth and creamy, adjusting sweetness with honey if desired.
3. Add ice cubes if a colder texture is preferred and blend again until well mixed.
4. Pour the smoothie into glasses, garnish with a few whole berries if desired, and enjoy the protein-packed and antioxidant-rich flavors of this berry spinach protein smoothie.

Preparation Time: Approximately 5-7 minutes

30. Green Tea Mango Smoothie

Ingredients:

- 1/2 cup mango chunks (fresh or frozen)
- 1/2 banana (fresh or frozen, sliced)
- 1/2 cup spinach leaves
- 1/2 cup brewed green tea (cooled)
- 1/2 cup Greek yogurt (unsweetened)

- 1 tablespoon honey (optional, adjust to taste)
- 1/2 cup unsweetened almond milk
- Ice cubes (optional)

Instructions:

1. Combine mango chunks, banana slices, spinach leaves, brewed green tea, Greek yogurt, honey (if using), and almond milk in a blender.
2. Blend until smooth and creamy, adjusting sweetness with honey if desired.
3. Add ice cubes if a colder texture is preferred and blend again until well mixed.
4. Pour the smoothie into glasses, garnish with a slice of mango if desired, and enjoy the refreshing and antioxidant-rich flavors of this green tea mango smoothie.

Preparation Time: Approximately 5-7 minutes

31. Creamy Papaya Coconut Smoothie

Ingredients:

- 1/2 cup papaya chunks (fresh or frozen)
- 1/2 banana (fresh or frozen, sliced)
- 1/4 cup coconut milk (unsweetened)
- 1/4 cup Greek yogurt (unsweetened)
- 1 tablespoon honey (optional, adjust to taste)

- 1/2 cup unsweetened almond milk
- Ice cubes (optional)

Instructions:

1. In a blender, combine papaya chunks, banana slices, coconut milk, Greek yogurt, honey (if using), and almond milk.
2. Blend until smooth and creamy, adjusting sweetness with honey if desired.
3. Add ice cubes if a colder texture is preferred and blend again until well mixed.
4. Pour the smoothie into glasses, garnish with a slice of papaya or a sprinkle of shredded coconut if desired, and enjoy the creamy and tropical flavors of this papaya coconut smoothie.

Preparation Time: Approximately 5-7 minutes

32. Blueberry Oatmeal Power Smoothie

Ingredients:

- 1/2 cup blueberries (fresh or frozen)
- 1/4 cup rolled oats
- 1/2 banana (fresh or frozen, sliced)
- 1/2 cup spinach leaves
- 1/2 cup Greek yogurt (unsweetened)
- 1 tablespoon honey (optional, adjust to taste)
- 1/2 cup unsweetened almond milk

- Ice cubes (optional)

Instructions:

1. Combine blueberries, rolled oats, banana slices, spinach leaves, Greek yogurt, honey (if using), and almond milk in a blender.
2. Blend until smooth and creamy, ensuring oats are well incorporated.
3. Add ice cubes if a colder texture is preferred and blend again until well mixed.
4. Pour the smoothie into glasses, garnish with a few blueberries or a sprinkle of oats if desired, and enjoy the nutritious and filling flavors of this blueberry oatmeal power smoothie.

Preparation Time: Approximately 5-7 minutes

33. Creamy Mango Pineapple Smoothie

Ingredients:

- 1/2 cup mango chunks (fresh or frozen)
- 1/2 cup pineapple chunks (fresh or frozen)
- 1/2 cup Greek yogurt (unsweetened)
- 1/4 cup coconut milk (unsweetened)
- 1 tablespoon honey (optional, adjust to taste)
- 1/2 cup unsweetened almond milk

- Ice cubes (optional)

Instructions:

1. In a blender, combine mango chunks, pineapple chunks, Greek yogurt, coconut milk, honey (if using), and almond milk.
2. Blend until smooth and creamy, adjusting sweetness with honey if desired.
3. Add ice cubes if a colder texture is preferred and blend again until well mixed.
4. Pour the smoothie into glasses, garnish with a pineapple slice or a sprinkle of shredded coconut if desired, and enjoy the tropical and creamy flavors of this mango pineapple smoothie.

Preparation Time: Approximately 5-7 minutes

34. Banana Berry Protein Smoothie

Ingredients:

- 1/2 banana (fresh or frozen, sliced)
- 1/2 cup mixed berries (strawberries, blueberries, raspberries)
- 1/2 cup spinach leaves
- 1/2 cup Greek yogurt (unsweetened)
- 1 scoop vanilla protein powder
- 1 tablespoon honey (optional, adjust to taste)

- 1/2 cup unsweetened almond milk
- Ice cubes (optional)

Instructions:

1. Combine banana slices, mixed berries, spinach leaves, Greek yogurt, protein powder, honey (if using), and almond milk in a blender.
2. Blend until smooth and creamy, adjusting sweetness with honey if desired.
3. Add ice cubes if a colder texture is preferred and blend again until well mixed.
4. Pour the smoothie into glasses, garnish with a few whole berries if desired, and enjoy the protein-packed and antioxidant-rich flavors of this banana berry protein smoothie.

Preparation Time: Approximately 5-7 minutes

35. Kiwi Coconut Lime Smoothie

Ingredients:

- 2 kiwis (peeled and sliced)
- 1/4 cup unsweetened shredded coconut
- Zest and juice of 1 lime
- 1/2 cup Greek yogurt (unsweetened)
- 1 tablespoon honey (optional, adjust to taste)

- 1/2 cup coconut water (unsweetened)
- Ice cubes (optional)

Instructions:

1. In a blender, combine kiwi slices, shredded coconut, lime zest, lime juice, Greek yogurt, honey (if using), and coconut water.
2. Blend until smooth and creamy, adjusting sweetness with honey if desired.
3. Add ice cubes if a colder texture is preferred and blend again until well mixed.
4. Pour the smoothie into glasses, garnish with a kiwi slice or a sprinkle of shredded coconut if desired, and enjoy the refreshing and tropical flavors of this kiwi coconut lime smoothie.

Preparation Time: Approximately 5-7 minutes

36. Pineapple Ginger Green Smoothie

Ingredients:

- 1/2 cup pineapple chunks (fresh or frozen)
- 1/2 banana (fresh or frozen, sliced)
- 1/2 cup spinach leaves
- 1/2 teaspoon freshly grated ginger
- 1/2 cup Greek yogurt (unsweetened)

- 1 tablespoon honey (optional, adjust to taste)
- 1/2 cup unsweetened almond milk
- Ice cubes (optional)

Instructions:

1. Combine pineapple chunks, banana slices, spinach leaves, freshly grated ginger, Greek yogurt, honey (if using), and almond milk in a blender.
2. Blend until smooth and creamy, adjusting sweetness with honey if desired.
3. Add ice cubes if a colder texture is preferred and blend again until well mixed.
4. Pour the smoothie into glasses, garnish with a pineapple slice or a sprinkle of grated ginger if desired, and enjoy the refreshing and zesty flavors of this pineapple ginger green smoothie.

Preparation Time: Approximately 5-7 minutes

37. Strawberry Banana Almond Smoothie

Ingredients:

- 1/2 cup strawberries (fresh or frozen)
- 1/2 banana (fresh or frozen, sliced)
- 1 tablespoon almond butter (unsweetened)
- 1/2 cup Greek yogurt (unsweetened)

- 1 tablespoon honey (optional, adjust to taste)
- 1/2 cup unsweetened almond milk
- Ice cubes (optional)

Instructions:

1. In a blender, combine strawberries, banana slices, almond butter, Greek yogurt, honey (if using), and almond milk.
2. Blend until smooth and creamy, adjusting sweetness with honey if desired.
3. Add ice cubes if a colder texture is preferred and blend again until well mixed.
4. Pour the smoothie into glasses, garnish with a strawberry on the rim if desired, and enjoy the delightful blend of strawberry, banana, and almond flavors in this smoothie.

Preparation Time: Approximately 5-7 minutes

38. Mango Avocado Green Smoothie

Ingredients:

- 1/2 cup mango chunks (fresh or frozen)
- 1/4 avocado (peeled and diced)
- 1/2 cup spinach leaves
- 1/2 cup cucumber (peeled and sliced)
- 1/2 cup Greek yogurt (unsweetened)
- 1 tablespoon honey (optional, adjust to taste)

- 1/2 cup coconut water (unsweetened)
- Ice cubes (optional)

Instructions:

1. Combine mango chunks, avocado chunks, spinach leaves, cucumber slices, Greek yogurt, honey (if using), and coconut water in a blender.
2. Blend until smooth and creamy, adjusting sweetness with honey if desired.
3. Add ice cubes if a colder texture is preferred and blend again until well mixed.
4. Pour the smoothie into glasses, garnish with a slice of mango or avocado if desired, and enjoy the creamy and nutrient-packed flavors of this mango avocado green smoothie.

Preparation Time: Approximately 5-7 minutes

39. Raspberry Coconut Chia Smoothies

Ingredients:

- 1/2 cup raspberries (fresh or frozen)
- 1/4 cup unsweetened shredded coconut
- 1 tablespoon chia seeds
- 1/2 cup Greek yogurt (unsweetened)
- 1 tablespoon honey (optional, adjust to taste)
- 1/2 cup unsweetened coconut milk

- Ice cubes (optional)

Instructions:

1. In a blender, combine raspberries, shredded coconut, chia seeds, Greek yogurt, honey (if using), and coconut milk.
2. Blend until smooth and creamy, adjusting sweetness with honey if desired.
3. Add ice cubes if a colder texture is preferred and blend again until well mixed.
4. Pour the smoothie into glasses, garnish with a sprinkle of shredded coconut if desired, and enjoy the refreshing and tropical flavors of this raspberry coconut chia smoothie.

Preparation Time: Approximately 5-7 minutes

40. Spinach Pineapple Mint Smoothie

Ingredients:

- 1/2 cup pineapple chunks (fresh or frozen)
- 1/2 cup spinach leaves
- 5-6 fresh mint leaves
- 1/2 cup Greek yogurt (unsweetened)
- 1 tablespoon honey (optional, adjust to taste)
- 1/2 cup unsweetened almond milk
- Ice cubes (optional)

Instructions:

1. Combine pineapple chunks, spinach leaves, fresh mint leaves, Greek yogurt, honey (if using), and almond milk in a blender.

2. Blend until smooth and creamy, adjusting sweetness with honey if desired.

3. Add ice cubes if a colder texture is preferred and blend again until well mixed.

4. Pour the smoothie into glasses, garnish with a sprig of mint if desired, and enjoy the refreshing and vibrant flavors of this spinach pineapple mint smoothie.

Preparation Time: Approximately 5-7 minutes

CONCLUSION

In conclusion, embracing smoothies for kidney health is a flavorful and health-conscious journey that combines nutrition and taste in a delicious concoction.

By focusing on kidney-friendly ingredients and mindful preparation, these smoothies offer a refreshing way to support renal function and overall well-being.

The principles of incorporating low-potassium and low-phosphorus fruits, along with hydrating bases like coconut water and almond milk, ensure a kidney-friendly balance.

The inclusion of nutrient-rich ingredients such as leafy greens, berries, and chia seeds provides essential vitamins, antioxidants, and fiber, contributing to a wholesome dietary approach.

Not only do these smoothies adhere to kidney health guidelines, but they also present a versatile and enjoyable means of staying hydrated.

The myriad of flavors, from tropical blends to berry-infused delights, caters to diverse tastes while accommodating the dietary restrictions often associated with kidney concerns.

Furthermore, the benefits of these smoothies extend beyond kidney support, encompassing improved hydration, boosted immune function, and enhanced digestion.

As a convenient and tasty option, these beverages stand as a valuable addition to a renal-friendly lifestyle.

By following the recommended guidelines, understanding the principles, and exploring the vast array of nutritious ingredients, individuals can craft smoothies that not only promote kidney health but also make each sip a pleasurable and health-conscious experience.

Smoothies for kidney health, with their delicious profiles and nutritional prowess, exemplify the fusion of wellness and indulgence in a glass, providing a satisfying and wholesome approach to caring for our kidneys.

www.ingramcontent.com/pod-product-compliance
Lightning Source LLC
Chambersburg PA
CBHW072000210526
45479CB00003B/1015